The Mysteries of Mumps, Measles and Rubella

The Inside Narrative of the Causes, Symptoms, and Treatment of These Deadly Diseases

Debbi Cooper

TABLE OF CONTENT

CHAPTER 7: PUBLIC HEALTH MEASURES AND COMMUNITY RESPONSES

CHAPTER 8: CONCLUSION: MOVING FORWARD TOGETHER

Introduction

In recent years, the comeback of vaccine-preventable illnesses has presented substantial difficulties to public health systems worldwide. Among these illnesses, mumps have emerged as a serious hazard, with periodic outbreaks happening in diverse areas. Understanding the dynamics of these outbreaks and the underlying causes is critical for successful disease control and preventive efforts.

Thank you for visiting "The Mysteries of Mumps, Measles, and Rubella." Through these pages, we will journey into the complicated network of these deadly foes to discover the secrets buried therein.

With each turn of the page, we trace the origins of these ancient diseases back through medical history. From the first reported outbreaks to the current problems of containment and eradication, we uncover the evolutionary processes that have formed and continue to affect the development of these illnesses.

But our investigation goes beyond historical interest; we address the grim facts of the current consequences of Mumps, Measles, and Rubella. We see the devastation caused by epidemics in communities worldwide and grapple with the human cost imposed by these tenacious opponents.

Despite the gloom, there is a glimmer of hope: the prospect of understanding and intervention. As we explore the complexities of Mumps, Measles, and Rubella, we arm ourselves with the information we need to confront these devious opponents. From recognizing early signs to adopting efficient treatment options, we have the skills to face these diseases head-on.

In "The Mysteries of Mumps, Measles, and Rubella," we go on a journey of enlightenment, motivated to uncover the secrets of these lethal illnesses. Let us together travel the labyrinth of science and medicine, guided by the light of knowledge and the will to unravel the mysteries that lie ahead.

Chapter 1: Understanding Recent Outbreaks

Mumps is a viral illness that causes salivary gland enlargement. It typically affects children and young people. Despite the availability of a safe and effective vaccine, mumps outbreaks persist, indicating gaps in vaccination coverage and protection. Recent outbreaks have been documented in various contexts, including schools, colleges, and communities, highlighting the need for increased surveillance and control measures.

One of the primary contributors to mumps epidemics is diminishing immunity among vaccinated persons. While the measles, mumps, and rubella (MMR) vaccination protects against mumps, immunity can wane over time, especially without booster doses. As a result, previously vaccinated people may become vulnerable to mumps infection, helping the virus spread among susceptible groups.

In addition to diminishing immunity, additional factors such as close contact in communal settings and foreign travel can contribute to the spread of mumps. Crowded locations, such as schools and dorms, create excellent conditions for transmission, allowing the virus to spread quickly among people in close contact. Furthermore, international travel can transfer mumps strains from outbreak-prone locations, resulting in localized clusters of infections in previously unaffected areas.

It is equally critical to note the impact vaccination reluctance and misinformation play in mumps epidemics. Despite overwhelming scientific evidence that vaccinations are safe and effective, misunderstandings and unwarranted fears continue, prompting some people to delay or avoid immunization for themselves or their children. This vaccination hesitation increases individual vulnerability to mumps and weakens communal immunity, increasing the likelihood of outbreaks.

Importance of Awareness and Prevention

Given the current mumps epidemic, raising awareness about the need for vaccination and preventative measures is critical. Vaccination is still the most effective technique for managing mumps and limiting its spread within communities. The MMR vaccination, which protects against measles, mumps, and rubella, is recommended for all children as part of their regular immunization plan. The MMR vaccination, given in two doses at ages 12-15 months and 4-6 years, provides long-term protection against mumps and other viral infections.

In addition to immunization, encouraging personal hygiene and implementing infection control measures can help lower the risk of mumps transmission. Encourage frequent hand washing, mask coughs and sneezes, and avoid close contact with sick people to help prevent the spread of mumps and other respiratory illnesses. Furthermore, anyone with symptoms of mumps, such as facial swelling and fever, should seek medical assistance immediately and avoid close contact with others to prevent further transmission.

Community participation and teamwork are also important parts of mumps preventive strategies. Health officials, healthcare professionals, educators, and community leaders all play important roles in spreading correct information about mumps and vaccinations, resolving misunderstandings, and increasing immunization rates. Communities can successfully lower the occurrence of mumps by working together to promote awareness and adopt preventative measures.

Recent mumps outbreaks have highlighted the continued problems faced by vaccine-preventable infections and the significance of proactive efforts to curb their spread. Communities can reduce the burden of mumps and protect public health by identifying the variables contributing to outbreaks and highlighting the necessity of vaccination and prevention initiatives. We can work together to create a future free of the threat of mumps epidemics by raising awareness, promoting immunization, and implementing infection control measures.

Chapter 2: Mumps, the Silent Threat

What is Mumps?

Mumps is a highly infectious viral infection caused by the mumps virus, which belongs to the Paramyxoviridae family. It primarily targets the salivary glands, causing severe swelling and inflammation. The virus spreads by respiratory droplets from an infected person, most commonly through coughing, sneezing, or close physical contact. Mumps can also spread indirectly by contact with infected surfaces or items.

After exposure to the virus, the incubation period normally lasts 12 to 25 days, during which infected persons may not display symptoms but can still spread the infection. When symptoms appear, the most distinctive hallmark of mumps is enlargement of the parotid glands, which are positioned on the sides of the face beneath the ears. This swelling gives affected people a distinct "chipmunk-like" look, with puffy cheeks and a bulging jaw.

In addition to parotitis (parotid gland swelling), mumps can induce fever, headache, muscular pains, exhaustion, and lack of appetite. Some people may have discomfort in swallowing or talking due to the enlarged glands pressing against adjacent tissues. While most mumps episodes recover without problems, serious complications can occur, particularly in older adolescents and adults.

Orchitis, or inflammation of the testicles in males, is one of the most dangerous consequences of mumps. It can cause discomfort, swelling, and infertility. Mumps in females can induce inflammation of the ovaries (oophoritis) or breast tissue (mastitis). Meningitis and encephalitis are rare but potentially life-threatening consequences of mumps.

Overview of the Recent Outbreak in New Jersey.

In recent months, New Jersey has seen an outbreak of mumps, with numerous confirmed cases in Hunterdon County. The outbreak has been traced down to a single family cluster with connections to international travel, demonstrating the global nature of infectious illness transmission. While the specific source of the outbreak may vary, foreign travel raises the danger of bringing contagious illnesses, such as mumps, from outbreak-prone areas.

The New Jersey Department of Health has aggressively monitored and responded to the mumps outbreak, collaborating with local health agencies to investigate cases, track down contacts, and implement control measures. Despite efforts to limit the virus, mumps epidemics can be difficult to manage, particularly in close-knit groups or areas with high population density.

The epidemic emphasizes the significance of maintaining high vaccination coverage rates to prevent the comeback of vaccine-preventable illnesses. Vaccination remains the most effective way to prevent mumps and reduce the danger of outbreaks. The measles, mumps, and rubella (MMR) vaccination, which protects against mumps, is recommended for all children as part of their immunization program.

Symptoms and Progression of Mumps

Mumps symptoms often appear in phases, beginning with nonspecific symptoms such as fever, headache, muscular pains, lethargy, and lack of appetite. During this stage, people may not recognize they are sick and may unwittingly spread the virus to others. The prodromal phase is followed by the development of parotitis, which is the primary symptom of mumps.

Parotitis often begins unilaterally (on one side) and can develop to include both parotid glands over several days. The swelling is frequently accompanied by discomfort and soreness, particularly while chewing or pressing on the afflicted glands. In extreme cases, swelling can spread to the neck and throat, making it difficult to swallow or breathe.

Mumps, in addition to parotitis, can cause difficulties in various organs and systems. Orchitis, or inflammation of the testicles, is one of the most prevalent problems among postpubertal boys, accounting for up to 30% of cases. Orchitis can cause significant discomfort, swelling, and soreness in the afflicted testicle and, in some cases, infertility.

Mumps in females can induce inflammation of the ovaries (oophoritis) or breast tissue (mastitis), resulting in stomach discomfort, fever, and breast soreness. While these consequences are less prevalent than orchitis, they can nonetheless cause substantial pain and necessitate medical attention.

Meningitis and encephalitis are rare yet significant neurological consequences of mumps that can develop simultaneously or after parotitis. Symptoms of mumps meningitis include headaches, neck stiffness, photophobia (light sensitivity), and altered mental state. Seizures, disorientation, and coma are some of the most severe symptoms of encephalitis, or brain inflammation.

The symptoms and course of mumps can vary greatly depending on age, immunological status, and underlying health issues. While most mumps infections are cured without difficulties, early detection and adequate therapy are critical to avoiding catastrophic outcomes and reducing the potential of transmission throughout communities. Vaccination is still the cornerstone of mumps prevention, providing safe and effective protection against this potentially dangerous viral illness.

Chapter 3: MMR Vaccine: Your Protection against Mumps

Importance of Vaccination

Vaccination is a successful public health measure for avoiding infectious illnesses and their sequelae. The measles, mumps, and rubella (MMR) vaccine exemplifies the effectiveness of immunization in controlling and eradicating vaccine-preventable diseases. The MMR vaccination protects against measles, mumps, and rubella for a long time by activating the immune response to these viruses, lowering the risk of illness and transmission among populations.

The necessity of mumps immunization cannot be emphasized, especially in light of recent outbreaks and the risk of catastrophic consequences. While mumps may appear to be a minor childhood sickness, it can cause serious problems, especially in teenagers and adults. Vaccinating people against mumps protects them against the infection's acute effects and long-term sequelae such as orchitis, meningitis, and encephalitis.

Furthermore, vaccination is critical in attaining herd immunity, which occurs when a large part of the population is immune to a disease, preventing it from spreading across the community. By boosting vaccine coverage, we can build a protective barrier that inhibits mumps transmission and lowers the danger of outbreaks.

This is especially crucial for safeguarding vulnerable groups, such as newborns too young to be vaccinated and those with weakened immune systems.

The MMR vaccine is safe, effective, and widely used as part of routine vaccination programs in many countries worldwide. Extensive scientific research and clinical studies have shown that vaccination is safe and effective in preventing mumps and other viral infections. Despite infrequent reports of side effects after vaccination, the benefits significantly exceed the dangers, and major consequences are uncommon.

The MMR vaccination protects against mumps and helps manage and eliminate measles and rubella, two more extremely common viral illnesses. By integrating both vaccinations into a single formulation, the MMR vaccine streamlines the vaccination procedure and increases immunization coverage rates. This integrated immunization strategy provides broad protection against various illnesses, requiring little healthcare resources and logistics.

In conclusion, mumps immunization with the MMR vaccine is critical for safeguarding people, communities, and public health systems from the burden of mumps outbreaks and sequelae. We can ensure everyone benefits from this life-saving strategy by increasing vaccine uptake and removing immunization obstacles.

A Two-Dose Schedule for Children and Adults

The MMR vaccine's recommended dosage regimen includes two doses to achieve optimum protection against measles, mumps, and rubella. The first dosage is usually given at 12 to 15 months, followed by a second dose between 4 and 6 years of age. This two-dose regimen is intended to provide strong and long-lasting protection against certain viral infections, reducing the likelihood of disease outbreaks and consequences.

The justification for the two-dose schedule stems from the vaccine's ability to stimulate an immunological response. While a single dose of the MMR vaccine elicits a significant immune response in most people, a second dose is required to establish appropriate levels of protection in those who may not have reacted well to the first immunization. The second vaccine strengthens and extends immunity, offering better protection against mumps and other infections.

The second dosage is intentionally timed to coincide with other normal children's immunizations, making it easier for parents and healthcare professionals to follow the recommended immunization schedule. We can guarantee that children are fully protected against measles, mumps, and rubella before exposure in educational settings by delivering the second dose before they reach school age.

In addition to the standard two-dose schedule for children, certain groups may require extra doses of the MMR vaccination to maintain immunity or respond to unique risks. Adolescents and adults who have not previously had two doses of the MMR vaccine or are at high risk of mumps infection should speak with their healthcare professionals to identify the best immunization regimen. Individuals going to mumps-infested areas or living in close quarters, such as college dorms or military barracks, may be affected.

Adherence to the two-dose schedule for the MMR vaccination is critical for establishing and maintaining protection against mumps and other viruses. By providing timely immunizations using established criteria, we can protect people of all ages from mumps' potentially devastating effects and help manage and eliminate vaccine-preventable infections.

Addressing Vaccination Hesitancy

Vaccine hesitancy, defined as a hesitation or unwillingness to vaccinate despite the availability of vaccines, is a major impediment to public health efforts to prevent infectious illnesses like mumps. While vaccination has helped to reduce the global burden of vaccine-preventable diseases, misunderstandings, disinformation, and mistrust of vaccines continue to drive skepticism and weaken immunization campaigns.

One of the key causes of vaccination reluctance is the dissemination of disinformation and falsehoods about vaccines, their safety, and effectiveness. Misinformation spread via social media, online forums, and anti-vaccine advocacy organizations can instill unjustified worries and anxieties in parents and caregivers, causing them to question the need and safety of vaccinating their children against mumps and other infections.

Another factor contributing to vaccine hesitation is the low disease risk, particularly for illnesses like mumps, which have grown less frequent due to effective immunization campaigns. Some people may underestimate the danger of mumps and its possible repercussions, putting the risks of vaccination ahead of the advantages of injection.

Furthermore, cultural, religious, and philosophical views might impact people's attitudes about vaccination and desire to follow prescribed immunization regimens. Cultural norms, social networks, and community views may all impact vaccine attitudes and influence healthcare decisions, including immunization against mumps and other infectious illnesses.

Addressing vaccine reluctance requires a diversified strategy that recognizes and responds to the various elements influencing people's attitudes about immunization. Effective techniques for dealing with vaccination reluctance include:

1. **Education and Communication**: Entail providing accurate, evidence-based information regarding immunizations, their safety, and their role in avoiding mumps and other infections. Health officials, practitioners, and community leaders must distribute clear,

understandable information to address common issues and misunderstandings.

2. **Building Trust and Confidence**: Developing trust between healthcare practitioners and patients via open, honest, and empathic communication. Listening to people's worries, answering their questions and fears, and giving individualized counseling can help them gain confidence in vaccination and reduce their concerns about vaccine safety and efficacy.

3. **Combating Disinformation**: Using focused communication, fact-checking activities, and social media involvement to dispel vaccination disinformation and misconceptions. Providing reputable sources of information and dispelling misleading claims enable people to make educated vaccination decisions based on scientific facts and professional advice.

4. **Community Engagement**: Working with communities, religious leaders, and cultural influencers to address the cultural and social issues that shape vaccination attitudes and behaviors. Vaccination messaging tailored to different cultural backgrounds and beliefs can increase community acceptability and support for immunization efforts against mumps and other infectious illnesses.

5. **Policy and Laws**: Enacting policies and regulations to improve vaccination mandates, increase vaccine availability and cost, and combat vaccine disinformation. Providing equal access to vaccinations and reducing obstacles to immunization can boost vaccine uptake and protect

communities from mumps outbreaks and other vaccine-preventable infections.

6. **Collaboration and Partnerships**: Encouraging collaboration among public health authorities, healthcare providers, community groups, and other stakeholders to coordinate immunization efforts and combat vaccine hesitancy at the local, national, and global levels. We can boost vaccination acceptability by developing personalized treatments and outreach methods based on our pooled experience and resources.

7. **Monitoring and Evaluation**: Include implementing effective surveillance systems to track vaccination coverage rates, vaccine-preventable illness incidence, and vaccine safety data. Continuous monitoring and assessment enable health officials to identify regions with low vaccination coverage, discover outbreaks early, and respond quickly with tailored treatments to combat the spread of mumps and other infectious illnesses.

8. **Empowering Healthcare Practitioners**: Providing healthcare practitioners with the information, skills, and resources they need to effectively communicate with patients about the benefits of vaccination and address vaccine hesitancy in clinical settings. Training in vaccine communication approaches, cultural competency, and effective risk communication can help doctors interact with patients and encourage immunization.

9. **Utilizing Digital Platforms**: Smartphone applications, and social media channels to deliver accurate vaccination

information and engage different audiences. Individuals may use interactive tools, instructional films, and online forums to access credible information, connect with healthcare experts, and make educated decisions regarding mumps vaccine and other infectious illnesses.

10. **Community-Led Initiatives**: We support grassroots and community-led initiatives to promote immunization and address vaccine reluctance within communities. Peer-to-peer education, community health ambassadors, and grassroots advocacy initiatives can successfully engage marginalized communities, foster trust, and enhance vaccination acceptability in difficult-to-reach groups.

Using a comprehensive and integrated strategy to tackling vaccine hesitancy, we may remove obstacles to vaccination and boost immunization efforts against mumps and other vaccine-preventable illnesses. By establishing trust, empowering individuals, and supporting evidence-based communication, we can guarantee everyone access to life-saving vaccinations while protecting communities from mumps epidemics and their associated problems. Together, we can create a healthier, more resilient society where vaccinations are recognized as critical instruments to safeguard public health and avoid infectious illnesses.

Chapter 4: Recognize and Respond to Symptoms

Identifying Early Signs of Mumps

Recognizing the early symptoms of mumps is critical for timely diagnosis and treatment. While mumps often begin with vague symptoms similar to other viral diseases, key distinguishing characteristics can help differentiate it from ordinary colds or flu. One of the first signs of mumps is a fever, frequently accompanied by headache, lethargy, and muscular pains. These flu-like symptoms may initially be minor and not indicate a mumps infection.

However, as the infection continues, distinctive mumps symptoms emerge, most notably enlargement of the parotid glands on the sides of the face below the ears. This swelling, known as parotitis, gives affected people a particular look, including puffy cheeks and a protruding jaw. Swelling can be unilateral (affecting only one side) or bilateral (affecting both sides) and ranges in degree from moderate to significant.

In addition to parotitis, mumps patients may suffer discomfort or soreness in the afflicted glands, particularly while chewing, swallowing, or applying pressure to the jaw. Some people may find it difficult to completely open their mouth owing to swelling, making eating, drinking, and speaking more uncomfortable. In extreme cases, swelling can spread to the neck and throat, causing pain and trouble breathing.

It is crucial to remember that not all mumps patients develop parotitis, and some may exhibit unusual or mild symptoms that do not immediately indicate mumps infection. In such circumstances, a high level of suspicion is required, especially if the patient has known mumps exposure or has recently been to a region where mumps outbreaks are occurring. Clinicians should consider mumps in the differential diagnosis of patients with compatible symptoms, especially during periods of elevated mumps activity in the community.

Seeking Prompt Medical Attention.

Individuals suspected of having mumps require prompt medical attention to obtain an accurate diagnosis, proper treatment, and advice on infection prevention measures. If you or someone you know has mumps-like symptoms, get medical attention right once, especially if the origin of the symptoms is unknown or if there are concerns about potential consequences.

When seeking medical assistance for suspected mumps, it is best to contact the healthcare provider's office or clinic and notify them of your symptoms and travel history, if any. This enables healthcare personnel to take adequate safeguards against mumps transmission to other patients and staff members. Healthcare institutions may have specific locations or methods for assessing and managing persons with probable mumps to reduce the risk of transmission.

During the medical assessment, healthcare experts will take a detailed history and physical examination to look for signs and symptoms of mumps infection. Diagnostic studies, including blood tests or viral swabs, may be used to confirm the diagnosis and rule out alternative explanations of the symptoms. Given the possibility of co-infection or exposure, healthcare practitioners may consider testing for other vaccine-preventable illnesses, such as measles and rubella, in cases of suspected mumps.

In addition to diagnostic tests, healthcare practitioners may prescribe supportive care measures to help patients recover from mumps. This may include advice for pain medication, water, relaxation, and isolation to prevent the illness from infecting others. Depending on the severity of their symptoms and sequelae, individuals suffering from mumps may require regular monitoring and follow-up treatment to ensure optimal infection management.

Individuals diagnosed with mumps should follow specified infection control measures to prevent the virus from spreading to others. This involves practicing excellent hand hygiene, concealing coughs and sneezes, avoiding close contact with others, and staying home from school or work until cleared by medical professionals. Individuals who take these steps can help protect their families, friends, and communities against the spread of mumps.

Complications and Long-Term Effects.

While mumps are usually a self-limiting condition that goes away independently, some people may develop problems or have long-term repercussions due to the virus.

Mumps complications can impact various organs and systems in the body, with minor to severe signs necessitating medical attention.

Orchitis, or inflammation of the testicles, is one of the most common consequences of mumps, affecting up to 30% of post-pubertal boys. Orchitis usually causes pain, swelling, and discomfort in one or both testicles, and it can be accompanied by fever and malaise. Extreme orchitis can cause testicular atrophy (shrinkage) and consequent reproductive problems. However, this is uncommon.

In addition to orchitis, mumps can induce reproductive system issues, such as oophoritis (ovary inflammation) in females and mastitis (breast tissue inflammation) in both sexes. If not recognized and treated swiftly, these consequences can include stomach discomfort, fever, and breast tenderness, as well as long-term reproductive health difficulties.

Mumps can damage the central nervous and reproductive systems, causing problems such as meningitis and encephalitis. Mumps meningitis, defined by inflammation of the protective membranes surrounding the brain and spinal cord, can induce headaches, neck stiffness, photophobia (sensitivity to light), and impaired mental state. While most cases of mumps meningitis recover without long-term consequences, severe or persistent inflammation can cause neurological issues.

Encephalitis, or brain inflammation, is a rare but dangerous mumps consequence that can cause convulsions, coma, and neurological impairments. Encephalitis can occur simultaneously with parotitis or as a later consequence of mumps infection. Mumps encephalitis, in extreme cases, can result in irreversible brain damage or even death, emphasizing the need for early detection and treatment of neurological symptoms.

In rare cases, mumps infection can cause pancreatitis (pancreatic inflammation), myocarditis (heart muscle inflammation), and sensorineural hearing loss. These consequences might occur concurrently with parotitis or weeks or months after the initial symptoms of the mumps have resolved. While most people recover completely from mumps without any long-term consequences, severe problems may need specialist medical care and continuing monitoring to avoid major morbidity and mortality.

Mumps' difficulties and long-term repercussions highlight the necessity of early detection, timely medical intervention, and proper infection control. Healthcare practitioners can reduce the likelihood of bad outcomes and guarantee optimum recovery for those who have had mumps by monitoring for symptoms of problems and providing supportive treatment when necessary. Furthermore, immunization against mumps with the MMR vaccine remains the most effective technique for avoiding mumps illness and its sequelae, emphasizing the need to maintain high vaccination rates in communities.

Chapter 5: Measles: Another Emerging Concern

Overview of Measles Outbreaks.

Measles, caused by the measles virus, is a highly infectious viral infection that remains a global public health hazard. Despite safe and effective vaccine availability, measles outbreaks continue, spurred by factors such as low vaccination rates, worldwide travel, and vaccine reluctance. Measles outbreaks can develop in areas with poor vaccination rates, resulting in clusters of cases and the potential for broad transmission.

In recent years, measles outbreaks have been documented in various locations, including areas with historically high vaccination rates. These outbreaks highlight the significance of maintaining high levels of community immunity through vaccination to prevent the resurgence of measles and its sequelae. The recurrence of measles outbreaks underlines the need for ongoing efforts to boost vaccination programs, improve monitoring systems, and remove obstacles to vaccine access and adoption.

Measles epidemics can have serious public health and economic consequences, putting a burden on healthcare systems, interrupting daily routines, and inflicting avoidable morbidity and mortality. In addition to the acute health repercussions, measles outbreaks can erode faith in vaccination efforts, promote vaccine reluctance, and impede progress toward global health organizations' measles eradication goals.

Measles outbreaks must be controlled and prevented through a comprehensive approach that includes vaccination, surveillance, outbreak response, and community participation. By implementing evidence-based policies to enhance vaccine coverage and minimize measles transmission, we can reduce the impact of outbreaks and protect vulnerable communities from the devastation caused by this avoidable illness.

Symptoms and Risks of Measles

Measles is distinguished by a characteristic rash, fever, and other systemic symptoms that usually appear 10 to 14 days after exposure to the virus. The earliest symptoms of measles are typically similar to those of a common cold or flu, such as fever, cough, runny nose, and red, watery eyes. However, the presence of specific distinguishing features can help distinguish measles from other respiratory illnesses.

One of the traditional indications of measles is the appearance of Koplik spots, which are little white dots on the inside of the cheeks early in the sickness. These patches are considered pathognomonic for measles and are an important diagnostic characteristic that can help detect the disease early. In addition to Koplik spots, those with measles may have a high temperature, lethargy, and lack of appetite, which can increase as the disease develops.

Measles' distinctive rash usually starts on the face and extends down to the trunk and limbs over many days. The rash is made up of tiny, red, elevated lesions that might mix to produce bigger regions of discoloration. As the rash progresses, afflicted persons may suffer severe itching and pain, disrupting everyday activities and sleep.

In addition to the acute symptoms of measles, the virus can cause problems, particularly in susceptible groups such as young children, pregnant women, and people with weaker immune systems. Common measles sequelae include otitis media (ear infections), pneumonia (lung inflammation), and diarrhea, which can increase dehydration and electrolyte imbalance.

More serious effects of measles include encephalitis (brain inflammation), which occurs in around 1 in every 1,000 cases and can cause irreversible neurological impairments or death. Measles can also depress the immune system, resulting in secondary bacterial illnesses such as pneumonia or sepsis, which can be fatal if not treated immediately with medicines.

Measles infection during pregnancy increases the chance of problems such as premature labor, low birth weight, and miscarriage. Measles infection during pregnancy can potentially cause congenital measles syndrome in neonates, which is marked by birth abnormalities, developmental delays, and other negative consequences.

Overall, the symptoms and hazards associated with measles underline the need for early detection, rapid medical care, and vaccination to prevent viral spread and reduce the impact of measles epidemics on public health and individual well-being.

Importance of Measles Vaccination

Vaccination against measles is the most effective method of avoiding illness and its sequelae. The measles vaccination, commonly given as part of the measles, mumps, and rubella (MMR) vaccine, provides long-term protection from measles and helps to manage and eliminate the illness.

The MMR vaccination is recommended for all children as part of standard immunization regimens, with the first dose being administered between the ages of 12 and 15 months and the second between the ages of 4 and 6. This two-dose regimen provides excellent measles protection and maintains high community immunity levels, preventing recurring measles outbreaks.

In addition to standard childhood vaccinations, certain groups may require extra doses of the MMR vaccine to establish measles protection. Adolescents and adults who have not previously had two doses of the MMR vaccine or are at a higher risk of measles exposure should speak with their doctors to identify the best immunization regimen.

The measles vaccine is safe, effective, and widely used in many nations' national immunization programs. Extensive scientific research and clinical studies have shown that the vaccination is secure and effective at avoiding measles infection and its sequelae.

Despite the known advantages of measles vaccination, vaccine hesitancy and misinformation impede vaccination efforts, resulting in low vaccination coverage rates in some populations. Addressing vaccine hesitancy involves a broad strategy that includes giving accurate information about vaccine safety and efficacy, addressing concerns and misconceptions, and engaging with communities to foster confidence in immunization programs.

Individuals and communities can be protected from measles outbreaks and their effects by boosting vaccination coverage rates and providing widespread access to measles immunization. Vaccination not only prevents sickness and saves deaths but also protects public health by lowering the total measles burden and reducing the chance of outbreaks in susceptible groups.

Furthermore, measles vaccination is crucial in worldwide efforts to eradicate and meet regional and global eradication targets established by organizations such as the World Health Organization (WHO) and the Centers for Disease Control and Prevention (CDC). Countries may get closer to eradicating measles by boosting vaccine coverage rates and implementing comprehensive immunization plans, providing a safer and healthier future for future generations.

In addition to individual and community benefits, measles vaccination has larger societal and economic implications by lowering healthcare expenses, limiting lost productivity, and lessening the social and economic consequences of measles epidemics. Governments and politicians may reap huge returns on investment by investing in measles vaccination programs and making immunization a public health priority.

To summarize, measles vaccination is critical to public health efforts to manage and prevent outbreaks, protect vulnerable people, and accomplish global measles eradication goals. We can successfully battle measles and its consequences by increasing vaccination coverage rates, tackling vaccine hesitancy, and enhancing immunization programs, protecting the health and well-being of individuals and communities worldwide. We can overcome the problems of measles via collaborative action and dedication to vaccination, creating a future in which measles is no longer a looming concern but rather a distant memory of a disease defeated by science and public health initiatives.

Chapter 6: Rubella: A Threat to Pregnant People.

Rubella, or German measles, is an infectious viral infection caused by the rubella virus. While rubella is usually a minor infection in children and adults, it can pose substantial hazards to pregnant women and their unborn children if caught during pregnancy. Understanding rubella symptoms is critical for early diagnosis and therapy of the infection.

Rubella symptoms frequently begin with a minor fever, followed by a characteristic rash that appears on the face and spreads to the trunk and limbs. The rash is made up of tiny, pink or red spots that might mix to produce bigger regions of discoloration. Unlike measles, rubella rash is lighter in color and less prominent. Rubella patients may also feel headache, sore throat, runny nose, and enlarged lymph nodes, notably behind the ears and at the base of the skull, in addition to the rash.

In many situations, rubella symptoms are minor and may go unreported or be confused with other viral infections. However, rubella can create difficulties, particularly in vulnerable groups such as pregnant women and those with weaker immune systems. As a result, healthcare personnel should retain a high level of suspicion for rubella, especially in pregnant women and people who may have been exposed to the virus.

Rubella infection during pregnancy can have devastating repercussions for both the pregnant woman and her unborn child. The major worry with rubella infection during pregnancy is the potential of congenital rubella syndrome (CRS), a group of birth malformations and developmental abnormalities caused by the rubella virus passing the placenta and infecting the growing fetus. The severity of CRS is determined by when rubella infection develops during pregnancy, with the first trimester having the highest risk of problems. During this important time of fetal development, the rubella virus can cause considerable harm to developing organs and tissues, resulting in a variety of birth abnormalities, including deafness, cataracts, heart problems, and developmental delays.

In addition to birth abnormalities, rubella infection during pregnancy increases the chance of miscarriage, stillbirth, and premature birth. Pregnant people who get rubella may also develop problems such as pneumonia, encephalitis (brain inflammation), and thrombocytopenia (low platelet count), which might increase the chance of negative consequences for both the mother and the baby.

Preventing rubella infection during pregnancy is critical for safeguarding maternal and fetal health while reducing the chance of CRS and other issues. Pregnant people should practice good hand hygiene, avoid close contact with people who are sick or have recently been vaccinated with live attenuated rubella vaccine, and seek medical attention if they develop rubella-like symptoms.

Prevention Strategies for Rubella

To prevent rubella infection, a multidisciplinary strategy is required, including vaccination, public health interventions, and education about the hazards of rubella during pregnancy. Vaccination against rubella with the measles, mumps, and rubella (MMR) vaccination is the most effective way to avoid rubella infection and sequelae. As part of standard immunization regimens, the MMR vaccination is safe, effective, and recommended for all persons, including children, adolescents, and adults.

The MMR vaccination is normally given in two doses, the first at 12 to 15 months and the second at 4 to 6 years of age. Establishing high vaccination coverage rates in the community can create herd immunity and lower the overall risk of rubella transmission among communities. Furthermore, catch-up vaccination programs aimed at vulnerable groups, such as the unvaccinated and those at high risk of infection, can help narrow immunity gaps and avoid rubella outbreaks.

In addition to immunization, public health strategies such as surveillance, outbreak response, and contact tracing are critical for avoiding rubella transmission and managing outbreaks. Rapid case detection and containment, along with targeted vaccination efforts in affected communities, can help to restrict rubella transmission and protect susceptible people from infection.

Education and awareness-raising initiatives are critical components of rubella prevention methods, especially for pregnant women and healthcare workers. Pregnant women should be taught about the hazards of rubella during pregnancy and the need to get vaccinated before becoming pregnant to ensure protection against rubella. Healthcare practitioners should be alert for rubella symptoms in pregnant patients and give appropriate counseling and care to avoid maternal and fetal problems.

Preventing rubella infection necessitates a coordinated and comprehensive strategy combining vaccination, public health measures, and education. We can safeguard pregnant women and their unborn kids from the tragic consequences of rubella infection while also contributing to improve maternal and child health outcomes by prioritizing rubella prevention initiatives and providing universal access to immunization.

Chapter 7: Public Health Measures and Community Responses

The Role of Health Departments in Outbreak Management

Public health departments are crucial in handling infectious epidemics like measles, mumps, rubella, and other vaccine-preventable disorders. These entities coordinate response activities, perform surveillance, and adopt control measures to prevent disease transmission within communities. One of the key tasks of health departments during epidemics is to undertake surveillance to track illness incidence and dissemination. This includes gathering and evaluating data on reported cases, determining transmission trends and patterns, and pinpointing high-risk individuals or geographic locations. Surveillance data informs public health actions and guides resource allocation to regions of highest need.

In addition to surveillance, health authorities are charged with researching outbreaks to ascertain the source of infection and probable transmission channels. This might include interviewing individuals and their contacts, performing environmental evaluations, and testing specimens to confirm the presence of the causal agent. By identifying the source of infection and understanding how the disease spreads, health authorities may apply targeted control measures to disrupt transmission and prevent disease spread.

Health departments also play an important role in establishing control measures to prevent epidemics and safeguard public health. This may involve instituting quarantine or isolation measures for those diagnosed with the disease, advising on infection management techniques, and advocating vaccination or post-exposure prophylaxis for those who are susceptible. Health departments may also work with other agencies and stakeholders to offer medical treatment, counseling, and social assistance to impacted individuals and communities.

Furthermore, health officials must communicate with the public and provide timely and accurate information regarding the outbreak. This may include sending public health alerts and advisories, holding media briefings, and disseminating information to the community through social media and other communication channels. Health departments may assist in establishing confidence by keeping the public informed and involved, encouraging compliance with control measures, and empowering individuals to take necessary action to protect themselves and their families.

Overall, health departments play an important role in epidemic management by performing surveillance, investigating cases, adopting control measures, and communicating with the general public. Their activities are critical in limiting the spread of infectious illnesses and ensuring community health and well-being.

Public Awareness Campaigns and Educational Initiatives

Public awareness campaigns and education programs are essential to preventing and managing infectious disease epidemics. These efforts attempt to raise public awareness of disease transmission, preventative techniques, and the significance of vaccination. One of the key purposes of public awareness campaigns is to educate the public about the signs and symptoms of infectious illnesses and the significance of getting medical attention as soon as possible if they develop symptoms that indicate infection. These initiatives empower individuals to detect and respond to sickness quickly, lowering the danger of future transmission throughout the community.

Public awareness campaigns promote preventative practices such as hand cleanliness, respiratory etiquette, and immunization to minimize illness risk and protect vulnerable groups. These initiatives address myths and misconceptions about vaccinations by providing information about recommended vaccination schedules, vaccine safety, and immunization benefits. In addition to educating the general population, awareness programs keep healthcare practitioners current on disease prevention and control practices. By offering training and resources to healthcare personnel, these efforts enhance clinical detection, diagnosis, and management of infectious illnesses, resulting in improved patient outcomes and more effective outbreak control.

Furthermore, public awareness initiatives work with communities to address cultural, socioeconomic, and behavioral aspects that influence illness transmission and control. By adapting messages and treatments to diverse communities' individual needs and preferences, these campaigns can improve the relevance and efficacy of public health messaging while encouraging community engagement in outbreak response activities.

Effective communication tactics are critical to the success of public awareness campaigns, including the use of clear, concise, and culturally relevant messages and numerous communication channels to reach varied audiences. These campaigns may increase their reach and impact using conventional media, social media, community collaborations, and grassroots outreach and develop a feeling of communal responsibility for disease prevention and control.

Public awareness campaigns and education programs are important in preventing and controlling infectious disease epidemics. By increasing awareness, encouraging preventative measures, and engaging communities, these projects allow people and communities to take action to protect themselves and others from infectious illnesses, resulting in healthier, more resilient communities.

Collaboration among Healthcare Providers and Communities.

Collaboration between healthcare practitioners and communities is critical to effective epidemic management and containment. Healthcare practitioners have an important role in identifying, treating, and preventing infectious illnesses, while communities work together to promote public health initiatives, assist afflicted persons, and improve access to healthcare.

Disease surveillance and reporting are critical components of healthcare provider-community partnerships. Healthcare professionals are frequently the initial point of contact for people seeking medical attention for infectious illnesses, and they play an important role in detecting and reporting suspected cases to public health authorities. Healthcare practitioners can drive public health response efforts by rapidly reporting cases and providing pertinent clinical and epidemiological information, resulting in early discovery and control of outbreaks.

In addition to surveillance and reporting, healthcare practitioners play an important role in providing medical care to those suffering from infectious illnesses. This includes giving patients prompt diagnosis, proper treatment, and supportive care, as well as applying infection control measures to prevent transmission in healthcare settings. By following established disease management standards and practices, healthcare practitioners may assist in reducing the impact of outbreaks on individual health and limit disease transmission in the community.

Furthermore, healthcare practitioners are reliable sources of information and direction for their patients and communities. Healthcare practitioners contribute to public education by giving accurate information regarding illness prevention, transmission, and treatment. They also play an important role in encouraging vaccination and other preventive measures that protect individuals and communities from infectious illnesses and lower the likelihood of outbreaks.

Partnerships with local public health agencies, community groups, schools, and other stakeholders help to promote collaboration between healthcare professionals and their communities. Healthcare providers and communities may improve their collective ability to prevent and manage infectious disease outbreaks by collaborating to design and implement coordinated response plans, sharing resources and knowledge, and engaging the public.

Effective collaboration between healthcare practitioners and communities is based on open communication, mutual respect, and common goals and objectives. By developing trust and cooperation between stakeholders, healthcare professionals and communities may respond to outbreaks more effectively, reduce the burden of infectious illnesses, and enhance overall health and well-being.

Finally, healthcare practitioners and communities must work together to manage and contain outbreaks effectively. Healthcare providers and communities can strengthen their collective capacity to prevent and control infectious disease outbreaks while also protecting individuals' and communities' health and well-being by collaborating to conduct surveillance, provide medical care, educate the public, and implement preventive measures.

Chapter 8: Conclusion: Moving Forward Together

Take Action to Protect Yourself and Your Community.

As we consider the problems posed by infectious disease epidemics, it becomes evident that taking action to safeguard ourselves and our communities is critical. Everyone must play a part in avoiding the spread of contagious illnesses and ensuring public health. We may reduce the risk of infection and improve the well-being of our communities by implementing simple yet effective preventative measures and remaining up to date on the latest suggestions and guidelines.

One of the most critical steps people can take to protect themselves and others is to practice basic hygiene, such as washing their hands often with soap and water, covering coughs and sneezes with a tissue or elbow, and avoiding close contact with ill people. These simple hygiene precautions can help minimize the spread of infectious illnesses, particularly respiratory viruses like measles and influenza, while also protecting susceptible people from infection.

Individuals should also remain current on prescribed vaccines to avoid vaccine-preventable infections, including measles, mumps, rubella, and flu. Vaccination is a safe and effective technique to increase immunity to infectious illnesses and protect individuals and communities from epidemics.

Individuals can lower the risk of disease transmission and contribute to herd immunity by ensuring that they and their families get vaccinated on approved schedules. This helps safeguard people who are unable to be vaccinated due to medical reasons.

Individuals may also help public health efforts to control and prevent infectious disease outbreaks by following public health recommendations and guidelines, assisting with contact tracing activities, and seeking medical care as soon as they acquire signs of illness. Individuals who are proactive in their attitude to health and well-being can play a critical role in decreasing the burden of infectious diseases on society while also increasing overall community health and resilience.

The Significance of Immunization in Mitigating Future Outbreaks.

Vaccination is a critical component of public health efforts to prevent infectious disease outbreaks and safeguard persons and communities from the devastation caused by vaccine-preventable illnesses. Vaccines have played an important role in lowering the global burden of contagious diseases, resulting in considerable reductions in morbidity, mortality, and disease-related consequences.

The value of immunization in averting future epidemics cannot be emphasized. Vaccines operate by activating the immune system to develop protective antibodies against particular pathogens like viruses and bacteria, preventing illness and lowering the risk of disease transmission throughout communities.

By reaching high vaccination coverage rates, we may create herd immunity and prevent epidemics from happening, even among susceptible individuals.

In addition to averting individual occurrences of disease, vaccination provides larger social advantages, such as lower healthcare costs, increased productivity, and improved general quality of life. Vaccination programs are low-cost public health initiatives that provide high returns on investment by avoiding sickness, disability, and early mortality while also decreasing the load on healthcare systems and economies.

Despite the known advantages of vaccination, vaccine hesitancy and misinformation continue to impede vaccination efforts, resulting in low vaccination coverage rates and outbreaks of vaccine-preventable illnesses. Addressing vaccine hesitancy necessitates a multimodal strategy that involves giving accurate information about vaccine safety and efficacy, addressing concerns and misconceptions, and fostering trust in vaccination programs via community participation and outreach.

Moving ahead, vaccination must be prioritized as a public health priority, with investments directed toward strengthening immunization systems, enhancing vaccine access and equality, and eliminating vaccination obstacles. Working together to promote vaccination and address vaccine hesitancy allows us to protect individuals and communities against infectious illnesses while also preventing future outbreaks, guaranteeing a better and more resilient future for everyone.

They Are Empowering Individuals To Be Informed And Safe.

Empowering people to be informed and safe is critical for effective epidemic management and containment. In an era of fast-emerging infectious disease concerns, being current on the most recent research, recommendations, and guidelines is critical for making educated health and well-being decisions. By providing individuals with correct information and resources, we can enable them to take proactive measures to protect themselves and their communities against infectious illnesses.

Individuals can be empowered via health education and promotion activities that give evidence-based information on illness prevention, transmission, and control. These campaigns can assist in promoting knowledge about the importance of hygienic habits, vaccinations, and other preventative measures, allowing people to make more educated decisions regarding their health.

Furthermore, public health authorities and healthcare practitioners play an important role in spreading timely and accurate information regarding infectious disease outbreaks, as well as advising on appropriate measures and precautions. Public health authorities may reach broad audiences and ensure that information is accessible and relevant to all sectors of the population by utilizing a variety of communication channels, including traditional media, social media, and community engagement.

Furthermore, enabling people to stay educated and safe necessitates cultivating a culture of trust, openness, and collaboration among public health officials, healthcare professionals, and communities. By engaging with communities, listening to their concerns, and involving them in decision-making processes, we may foster trust and establish partnerships, which are critical for effective outbreak response and control. Empowering individuals to be aware and secure is a shared duty that necessitates joint effort and cross-sector collaboration. We can create a safer and healthier future for everyone by collaborating to promote health literacy, give access to correct information, and assist individuals in making healthy choices.

To summarize, taking action to protect ourselves and our communities, emphasizing vaccination as a cornerstone of disease prevention, and enabling individuals to be educated and safe are critical for effective outbreak management and control. Working together and adopting proactive actions to avoid infectious illnesses allows us to develop healthier, more resilient communities and a brighter future for future generations.

www.ingramcontent.com/pod-product-compliance
Lightning Source LLC
Chambersburg PA
CBHW070741260726
48660CB00007B/2929